FITNESS REBOOT

Sculpting Your Body in 60 Days

Sam Thomas

Table of Contents

INTRODUCTION

"Fitness Reboot: Sculpting Your Body in 60 Days" is a transformative guide that empowers individuals to embark on a comprehensive wellness journey, reshaping their bodies and revitalizing their lives in just two months. Authored with expertise and a profound understanding of fitness, this book serves as an invaluable companion for those seeking a potent, time-bound transformation.

In a world where health often takes a backseat to demanding schedules and sedentary lifestyles, "Fitness Reboot" emerges as a beacon of hope. This book isn't merely about quick fixes; it's about instilling lasting habits that foster physical and mental well-being. The author draws on cutting-edge exercise science, nutritional insights, and motivational strategies to craft a holistic approach.

Readers are invited to commit themselves to a 60-day program that merges workout routines, dietary guidelines, and mindfulness practices. The book's meticulously designed fitness regimens cater to various fitness levels, ensuring that both beginners and experienced individuals can progress effectively. Moreover, the nutritional guidance offered is practical and adaptable, promoting a sustainable relationship with food.

More than a physical transformation, "Fitness Reboot" underscores the significance of mental resilience gained through self-discipline and perseverance. As readers sculpt their bodies, they simultaneously cultivate inner strength. In a mere 200 pages, this introduction only hints at the comprehensive wisdom that "Fitness Reboot: Sculpting Your Body in 60 Days" contains, awaiting discovery by those ready to embrace positive change.

CHAPTER ONE

The Foundation: Understanding Your Goals and Body

In the pursuit of fitness and body transformation, setting the right foundation is essential. This chapter serves as the compass that guides readers through the initial stages of their fitness journey, emphasizing the significance of clear objectives and a comprehensive understanding of their bodies. By gaining insights into individual body types, realistic goal-setting, and the interplay between exercise and nutrition, readers will lay the groundwork for a successful 60-day fitness reboot.

Setting Clear Fitness Objectives

Before embarking on any fitness journey, it's crucial to define your objectives. Whether you're aiming to lose weight, gain muscle, increase endurance, or improve overall health, setting clear and achievable goals is the first step. Realistic goal-setting prevents frustration and disappointment, ensuring that your expectations align with the time and effort you're willing to invest. It's important to establish both short-term and long-term goals, allowing for a sense of accomplishment along the way while maintaining focus on the ultimate transformation.

Understanding Body Types: Ectomorphs, Mesomorphs, and Endomorphs

One size does not fit all in the realm of fitness. Our bodies are unique, and they respond differently to exercise and nutrition. Understanding your body type can provide valuable insights into how you should structure your fitness program. There are three primary body types: ectomorphs, mesomorphs, and endomorphs.

- Ectomorphs: Ectomorphs typically have a lean and slender build with fast metabolisms. They may find it challenging to gain muscle mass but are often more suited for endurance activities. Ectomorphs should focus on nutrient-dense meals and strength training to promote muscle growth.

- Mesomorphs: Mesomorphs are naturally muscular and athletic, with a propensity to gain muscle and lose fat relatively easily. They excel in a wide range of physical activities and can benefit from a balanced combination of strength training and cardiovascular exercises.

- Endomorphs: Endomorphs tend to carry more body fat and have a slower metabolism. They might find it more difficult to shed excess weight but can build significant muscle mass. Endomorphs benefit from a well-rounded fitness regimen that includes both strength training and calorie-controlled nutrition.

The Role of Realistic Goal-Setting

When it comes to fitness goals, setting attainable targets is essential for maintaining motivation and adherence. Unrealistic goals, such as expecting dramatic changes within a short time frame, can lead to disappointment and even burnout. Instead, focus on incremental progress and celebrate small victories along the way. For instance, if your goal is to lose a certain amount of weight, break it down into monthly or weekly milestones.

The Synergy of Exercise and Nutrition

Exercise and nutrition are two pillars that support any fitness journey. The right combination of these elements can accelerate progress and enhance results. Engaging in regular physical activity not only burns calories but also boosts metabolism, improves cardiovascular health, and promotes muscle growth. Strength training, cardiovascular exercises, and flexibility routines each play a role in a well-rounded fitness program.

However, even the most rigorous exercise routine can be undermined by poor nutrition. The saying "you can't out-train a bad diet" holds true. Fueling your body with the right nutrients is crucial for energy, recovery, and achieving your fitness goals. Protein, carbohydrates, fats, vitamins, and minerals all contribute to overall well-being and performance. Tracking your macronutrient intake and adopting a balanced approach to eating can optimize your results.

Mindset and the Long-Term Approach

As you embark on your fitness journey, cultivating the right mindset is paramount. Patience, consistency, and dedication are virtues that will serve you well. Rapid transformations often come with unsustainable practices, leading to a cycle of yo-yo dieting and fluctuating fitness levels. Instead, embrace the idea of a long-term approach. The 60-day program outlined in this book is just the beginning. It's a stepping stone toward a lifestyle that prioritizes health and wellness.

In conclusion, the foundation you lay at the start of your fitness journey will significantly impact your results. By setting clear objectives, understanding your body type, and recognizing the synergy between exercise and nutrition, you're primed for success. Remember that fitness is a personalized journey, and progress may vary. Stay committed, stay motivated, and stay true to your unique path toward transformation. The next chapters will delve deeper into the practical aspects of implementing this foundation, guiding you through the 60-day fitness reboot that awaits.

CHAPTER TWO
Day 1-15: Jumpstarting Your Transformation

The first 15 days of a fitness journey are often the most pivotal. This chapter is designed to provide you with the tools and guidance needed to kickstart your transformation on the right foot. As you embark on this initial phase, you'll be focusing on building momentum, establishing a consistent routine, and embracing fundamental exercises that target your entire body. With a combination of full-body workouts, cardio routines, and mindful dietary adjustments, these two weeks will set the tone for the rest of your 60-day journey.

Creating a Structured Workout Plan

A structured workout plan is essential during the jumpstart phase. The goal is to engage your entire body while gradually increasing the intensity of your exercises. Incorporating both strength training and cardiovascular workouts ensures a balanced approach to fitness. A sample workout plan for the first 15 days could look like this:

Day 1-5:
- Full-Body Strength Training: Focus on compound exercises that engage multiple muscle groups.

Squats, push-ups, lunges, and planks are excellent choices. Perform 3 sets of 10-12 repetitions each.

**Day 6-10:
- Cardiovascular Workouts: Incorporate 20-30 minutes of moderate-intensity cardio exercises such as brisk walking, jogging, or cycling. Gradually increase the duration and intensity over these five days.

Day 11-15:
- Full-Body Circuit: Combine strength and cardio in a circuit format. Perform each exercise for 45 seconds, followed by a 15-second rest. Repeat the circuit 3 times.

Exercises can include:
- Jump squats
- Push-ups
- Mountain climbers
- Dumbbell rows
- Burpees

Cardiovascular Routine and Its Importance

Cardiovascular exercise is a cornerstone of any fitness program. It enhances cardiovascular health, burns calories, and boosts endurance. During the initial 15 days, your cardiovascular routine will help improve your stamina and set the foundation for more intense workouts in the weeks to come.

Simple Dietary Adjustments

In addition to exercise, small dietary adjustments can have a significant impact on your progress. Focus on nutrient-dense foods that fuel your body and support your workouts. While it's important to tailor your nutrition to your individual needs and goals, here are some general guidelines for the first 15 days:

- Hydration: Drink plenty of water throughout the day to stay hydrated. Proper hydration supports energy levels and aids in recovery.

- Protein Intake: Include lean protein sources such as chicken, fish, tofu, and legumes in your meals. Protein is essential for muscle repair and growth.

- Complex Carbohydrates: Opt for whole grains like brown rice, quinoa, and oats. Complex carbohydrates provide sustained energy for your workouts.

- Healthy Fats: Incorporate sources of healthy fats such as avocados, nuts, seeds, and olive oil. These fats support overall health and satiety.

- Portion Control: Pay attention to portion sizes to avoid overeating. Listen to your body's hunger and fullness cues.

Overcoming Initial Challenges and Staying Motivated

The early days of any fitness journey can be challenging. You might encounter muscle soreness, fatigue, or even doubts about your ability to keep going. It's important to remember that these challenges are normal and temporary. Here are strategies to help you overcome them and stay motivated:

- Set Short-Term Goals: Break down your larger fitness goal into smaller, achievable milestones. Celebrate these victories to boost your motivation.

- Embrace the Process: Transformation takes time. Focus on the positive changes you're making in your daily routine rather than solely on the end result.

- Listen to Your Body: Pay attention to how your body feels. If you're experiencing excessive tiredness or fatigue, don't hesitate to scale back temporarily.

- Incorporate Variety: Keep your workouts interesting by introducing new exercises and routines. Variety prevents boredom and plateaus.

- Track Your Progress: Keep a workout journal or use a fitness app to track your workouts, nutrition, and how you're feeling. Seeing your progress can be incredibly motivating.

In conclusion, the first 15 days of your fitness journey are all about laying the groundwork for success. By following a structured workout plan, incorporating cardiovascular exercise, making simple dietary adjustments, and overcoming initial challenges, you'll build the momentum needed to carry you through the remainder of the 60-day program. Remember that every step forward, no matter how small, is a step toward achieving your goals. Stay committed, stay motivated, and stay excited about the transformative journey ahead.

CHAPTER THREE

Nutrition Essentials: Fueling Your Fitness Journey

In the intricate tapestry of achieving fitness goals, nutrition forms the vibrant thread that weaves together strength, endurance, and overall well-being. This chapter is a comprehensive exploration of the fundamental role that nutrition plays in your fitness journey. From understanding macronutrient ratios to practicing portion control, optimizing meal timing, and embracing hydration, you'll discover how to nourish your body for sustained energy, muscle development, and long-term success. As we delve into this chapter, we'll debunk common misconceptions surrounding diets and unveil a balanced approach to eating that harmonizes with your body's unique needs.

Understanding Macronutrient Ratios

Macronutrients—protein, carbohydrates, and fats—are the building blocks of a balanced diet that supports your fitness goals. Each macronutrient serves a specific purpose in your body:

- Protein: The foundation of muscle repair and growth. It's essential for anyone seeking to build lean muscle mass or recover from intense workouts.

- Carbohydrates: The primary source of energy for your body. Complex carbohydrates provide sustained energy for workouts and daily activities.

- Fats: Crucial for overall health, hormone production, and energy storage. Healthy fats support cellular function and provide a sense of satiety.

While individual needs vary, a balanced ratio to consider is 40% carbohydrates, 30% protein, and 30% healthy fats. However, these ratios can be adjusted based on your goals and preferences. For example, if you're focusing on muscle gain, you might increase your protein intake slightly.

Portion Control and Mindful Eating

Portion control is a cornerstone of effective nutrition. Even the healthiest foods can contribute to weight gain if consumed excessively. Practice mindful eating by paying attention to hunger and fullness cues. A simple approach is to use your hand as a guide:

- Protein: A portion size is roughly the size of your palm.

- Carbohydrates: A portion size is about the size of your clenched fist.
- Fats: A portion size is approximately the size of your thumb.

Remember that these are general guidelines and can be adjusted based on your energy expenditure and goals. Listen to your body, eat when you're hungry, and stop when you're satisfied.

Strategic Meal Timing

Meal timing plays a role in optimizing your energy levels, performance, and recovery. Here are some key principles to consider:

- Pre-Workout Nutrition: Consume a balanced meal containing carbohydrates and protein about 1-2 hours before your workout. This provides fuel for your workout and supports muscle preservation.

- Post-Workout Nutrition: Within 1-2 hours after your workout, consume a meal rich in protein and carbohydrates to aid in muscle recovery and replenish glycogen stores.

- Balanced Meals: Aim for regular, balanced meals throughout the day to maintain steady energy levels and prevent overeating later on.

Hydration: The Unsung Hero

Hydration is often underestimated in its role within the realm of fitness. Staying adequately hydrated is crucial for numerous physiological functions, including digestion, circulation, and temperature regulation. When you're exercising, your body loses fluids through sweat, making hydration even more vital.

- Pre-Workout Hydration: Drink water before your workout to ensure that you're adequately hydrated. Aim to consume around 16-20 ounces of water an hour before exercising.

- During-Workout Hydration: Sip water throughout your workout, especially if it's intense or prolonged. Listen to your body and drink when you feel the need.

- Post-Workout Hydration: Rehydrate after your workout to replace fluids lost through sweat. Water is a good option, but if you've had an intense workout, consider a sports drink that contains electrolytes.

Debunking Diet Myths

The world of nutrition is often muddled with conflicting advice and fad diets. It's important to discern fact from fiction to make informed choices. Here are some common diet myths debunked:

- Myth: Carbs Are Bad: Carbohydrates are not the enemy. Complex carbohydrates provide essential energy for your body. Focus on whole grains, fruits, and vegetables.

- Myth: No Fat Means Better Health: Healthy fats are essential for various bodily functions. Opt for sources like avocados, nuts, seeds, and olive oil.

- Myth: Skipping Meals Aids Weight Loss: Skipping meals can actually hinder weight loss by slowing down your metabolism and leading to overeating later. Regular, balanced meals are crucial.

Embracing Balance for Sustainable Progress

Amid the plethora of diet trends, it's essential to adopt an approach that is both effective and sustainable. Instead of fixating on rigid rules, embrace balance. Incorporate a variety of nutrient-rich foods into your diet to ensure that you're getting all the vitamins, minerals, and nutrients your body needs. Be open to trying new foods and finding what works best for your unique body and lifestyle.

In conclusion, nutrition is the bedrock of your fitness journey. By understanding macronutrient ratios, practicing portion control, optimizing meal timing, and embracing hydration, you'll nourish your body for peak performance and lasting success. Dispelling diet myths and adopting a balanced approach will empower you to make choices that align with your goals and promote your overall well-being. As you continue your 60-day transformation, remember that every meal is an opportunity to fuel your body's potential and thrive in your pursuit of fitness excellence.

CHAPTER FOUR

Day 16-30: Sculpting and Shaping

As you transition into the second phase of your 60-day fitness journey, the spotlight shifts to sculpting and shaping your body with precision. This chapter is a comprehensive guide to this pivotal phase, where your focus will be on targeted exercises that enhance muscle definition and toning. Through detailed workout plans, you'll engage specific muscle groups to create a harmonious balance of strength and aesthetics. Additionally, this chapter introduces advanced cardio techniques that amplify your fat-burning potential, propelling you further along the path to transformation.

The Significance of Targeted Exercises

While full-body workouts lay the foundation for fitness, targeted exercises refine that foundation, allowing you to shape your body according to your goals. Whether you're aiming for more defined abs, sculpted arms, or a stronger back, these targeted exercises are tailored to cater to specific muscle groups, promoting symmetry and balance.

Day 16-20: Lower Body Sculpting
- Squats: Perform various squat variations, such as goblet squats, sumo squats, and Bulgarian split squats, to engage your quadriceps, hamstrings, and glutes.

- Lunges: Incorporate forward lunges, reverse lunges, and lateral lunges to target your leg muscles from different angles.

- Deadlifts: Engage your hamstrings, glutes, and lower back with deadlift variations, such as Romanian deadlifts and stiff-legged deadlifts.

Day 21-25: Upper Body Definition
- Push-Ups: Focus on different push-up variations—standard, incline, and decline—to sculpt your chest, shoulders, and triceps.

- Pull-Ups or Rows: Engage your back, biceps, and shoulders with pull-ups or bent-over rows using dumbbells or resistance bands.

- Dips: Tone your triceps and chest with dips, using parallel bars or a sturdy surface.

Day 26-30: Core Strengthening

- Planks: Perform various plank variations—forearm planks, side planks, and plank jacks—to strengthen your core muscles.

- Russian Twists: Engage your obliques with Russian twists, using a medicine ball or weight.

- Leg Raises: Target your lower abdominal muscles with leg raises, either lying down or hanging from a bar.

Elevating Fat-Burning Potential with Advanced Cardio Techniques

Cardiovascular exercise is an indispensable component of any fitness program, and during the sculpting phase, advanced cardio techniques can amplify your fat-burning potential and boost your endurance.

High-Intensity Interval Training (HIIT): HIIT involves alternating between short bursts of intense exercise and periods of lower-intensity recovery. This approach challenges your cardiovascular system and accelerates calorie burning, even after the workout is done.

Tabata Training: Tabata is a form of HIIT that consists of 20 seconds of all-out effort followed by 10 seconds of rest, repeated for 4 minutes. This protocol is time-efficient and remarkably effective at increasing cardiovascular fitness.

Incorporating Active Rest: During your cardio sessions, integrate active rest periods that involve low-intensity exercises like jogging in place or doing jumping jacks. This keeps your heart rate elevated while allowing your muscles to recover slightly.

Nutrition to Support Sculpting and Shaping

As you intensify your workouts and focus on targeted exercises, proper nutrition remains paramount. Fuel your body with the right nutrients to support muscle recovery, growth, and fat loss.

Protein Intake: Maintain an adequate intake of protein to facilitate muscle repair and growth. Lean protein sources such as chicken, turkey, fish, and plant-based options are excellent choices.

Balanced Carbohydrates: Complex carbohydrates like sweet potatoes, quinoa, and brown rice provide sustained energy for your workouts and aid in recovery.

Healthy Fats: Continue to incorporate sources of healthy fats, such as avocados, nuts, and olive oil, for overall health and satiety.

Hydration: With increased physical activity, hydration is crucial. Consume water before, during, and after your workouts to stay adequately hydrated.

Recovery and Rest

As the intensity of your workouts increases, prioritizing recovery becomes even more essential. Ensure you're getting adequate sleep to support muscle recovery and overall well-being. Incorporate dynamic stretching, foam rolling, and yoga to enhance flexibility and reduce muscle soreness.

Staying Motivated and Adapting

Challenges and plateaus are natural as you progress through this phase. To maintain motivation:

- Set new goals: Whether it's increasing the weight you lift or mastering a challenging exercise, setting new goals keeps you engaged.
- Monitor progress: Track your improvements in strength, endurance, and physique to stay motivated.

- Embrace variety: Continuously introduce new exercises and techniques to prevent boredom and stimulate progress.

In conclusion, the second phase of your fitness journey is about refining your physique through targeted exercises and advanced cardio techniques. By engaging specific muscle groups and elevating your cardiovascular endurance, you're sculpting and shaping your body to align with your goals. With proper nutrition, adequate rest, and a motivated mindset, you're poised to make significant strides in the pursuit of your fitness transformation. As you enter the next phase of your 60-day journey, remember that each workout is a step toward achieving the sculpted and defined physique you're working hard to attain.

CHAPTER FIVE

Mind and Body Synergy: Incorporating Mindfulness

In the pursuit of fitness and wellness, the connection between mind and body is a fundamental aspect often overlooked. This chapter explores the transformative power of mindfulness practices, unveiling their profound impact on your fitness journey. By incorporating techniques such as meditation, visualization, and stress reduction, you'll cultivate a positive mindset that not only enhances motivation but also reduces stress-related setbacks. Through this chapter, you'll discover how the synergy between your mental and physical well-being can elevate your performance, adherence to the program, and overall sense of fulfillment.

The Power of Mindfulness

Mindfulness is the practice of being fully present and aware in the current moment, without judgment. It provides a mental toolkit that empowers you to navigate challenges, stressors, and setbacks with resilience. When applied to your fitness journey, mindfulness can be a transformative force that fosters sustainable progress and holistic well-being.

Meditation for Mental Clarity

Meditation is a cornerstone of mindfulness, offering a refuge of tranquility in our fast-paced lives. Just a few minutes of daily meditation can quiet the mind, reduce stress, and enhance focus. To incorporate meditation into your routine:

- Find a quiet space where you won't be disturbed.
- Sit comfortably with a straight spine and close your eyes.
- Focus on your breath, observing its natural rhythm.
- When thoughts arise, gently bring your attention back to your breath.

Visualization for Success

Visualization is a powerful tool that harnesses the mind's ability to create positive outcomes. By vividly imagining yourself achieving your fitness goals, you're priming your subconscious mind for success. Incorporate visualization into your routine:

- Find a quiet space and sit or lie down in a comfortable position.
- Close your eyes and envision yourself successfully completing your workouts, feeling strong and confident.

- Imagine the sensations, sights, and sounds associated with your fitness journey.

Stress Reduction Techniques

Stress is a common adversary in any transformative journey. However, how you respond to stress greatly influences your overall well-being. Incorporate stress reduction techniques to navigate challenges with grace:

- Deep Breathing: When stress arises, take slow, deep breaths. Inhale for a count of four, hold for four, and exhale for four. This calms the nervous system and reduces stress hormones.

- Progressive Muscle Relaxation: This technique involves tensing and then relaxing each muscle group in your body. It's an effective way to release physical tension caused by stress.

- Mindful Movement: Engage in mindful activities like yoga or tai chi. These practices combine movement with breath, enhancing body awareness and reducing stress.

The Mind-Body Connection in Fitness

The mind-body connection is not a one-way street; it's a dynamic interplay. A positive mindset can enhance your physical performance, while physical activity can boost your mood and reduce stress. Here's how:

- Motivation and Mindset: A positive mindset enhances motivation. When you approach workouts with enthusiasm and optimism, you're more likely to give your best effort.

- Stress Reduction: Physical activity releases endorphins—feel-good hormones—that combat stress and improve mood.

- Coping with Setbacks: Mindfulness equips you with tools to navigate setbacks. Instead of feeling defeated by a missed workout or a slip in nutrition, you can respond with self-compassion and resilience.

- Enhanced Adherence: Mindfulness helps you stay present in your fitness journey. This prevents you from getting overwhelmed by long-term goals and encourages consistent adherence to daily practices.

Creating a Mindful Routine

Incorporating mindfulness into your daily routine doesn't have to be time-consuming. Start with a few minutes each day and gradually build from there. Here's a sample routine:

- Morning: Begin your day with a brief meditation session to set a positive tone for the day ahead.

- Midday: Take a short break to practice deep breathing or engage in a quick visualization exercise.

- Evening: Wind down with a longer meditation session to release any tension from the day.

The Holistic Journey

As you integrate mindfulness into your fitness journey, remember that it's not just about achieving physical goals. It's about cultivating a sense of well-being, balance, and self-awareness. Embrace the ups and downs of your journey with equanimity, and recognize that every step forward—mindful and intentional—is a triumph.

In conclusion, the synergy between mind and body is a potent catalyst for transformative change. By incorporating mindfulness practices like meditation, visualization, and stress reduction, you're nurturing a positive mindset that enhances motivation, reduces stress-related setbacks, and fosters adherence to the program. The harmonious interplay between mental and physical well-being empowers you to not only sculpt your body but also elevate your overall quality of life. As you proceed with your 60-day journey, carry the wisdom of mindfulness with you, allowing it to illuminate each step on the path to a healthier, happier you.

CHAPTER SIX

Day 31-45: Power and Endurance

As you reach the mid-point of your 60-day fitness transformation, your body is primed for the next level of challenges. This chapter marks a significant shift in focus towards enhancing power and endurance. With the foundational strength in place, the aim is to push your limits, optimize performance, and elevate your fitness to new heights. Through the incorporation of higher intensity workouts, circuit training, interval workouts, and progressive resistance techniques, you'll cultivate power and endurance that propel you towards your goals. This chapter also underscores the crucial role of rest and recovery in sustaining your progress during this rigorous phase.

Harnessing Higher Intensity Workouts

Higher intensity workouts are the crucible in which power and endurance are forged. These workouts push your limits, challenge your cardiovascular system, and accelerate progress. The mid-point of your fitness journey is the ideal juncture to introduce these workouts, as your body has acclimated to the initial phases.

Circuit Training for Total-body Intensity

Circuit training combines strength and cardio exercises in rapid succession, creating a potent full-body workout. This approach maximizes calorie burn, boosts cardiovascular fitness, and enhances muscular endurance. Design a circuit that includes:

- Strength Moves: Incorporate compound movements like squats, lunges, push-ups, and rows.

- Cardio Bursts: Include cardio exercises like jumping jacks, high knees, or burpees to elevate your heart rate.

- Recovery Periods: Intersperse short rest intervals between exercises to maintain intensity.

Complete the circuit 2-3 times with minimal rest between sets.

Interval Workouts for Enhanced Endurance

Interval training involves alternating between high-intensity bursts and periods of low-intensity recovery. This method improves cardiovascular fitness, burns more calories, and challenges your body to adapt to varying levels of intensity.

Sample Interval Workout:
- Warm up with 5-10 minutes of light cardio.
- Alternate between 1 minute of all-out effort (sprinting, high knees) and 2 minutes of low-intensity recovery (walking or slow jogging).
- Repeat the cycle for 20-30 minutes.
- Cool down with 5-10 minutes of stretching.

Progressive Resistance Techniques

Progressive resistance techniques are paramount for building strength and power. These techniques challenge your muscles by progressively increasing resistance or intensity over time.

- Pyramid Sets: Start with light weights and gradually increase the weight with each set while decreasing the repetitions.

- Drop Sets: Perform an exercise with a heavy weight until failure, then immediately reduce the weight and continue until failure again.

- Supersets: Combine two exercises targeting different muscle groups with minimal rest in between. This technique increases intensity and efficiency.

Rest and Recovery: The Cornerstone of Progress

In the pursuit of power and endurance, rest and recovery are not mere luxuries; they're essential components of your progress. Adequate rest allows your muscles to recover and rebuild, preventing overtraining and injury.

Sleep: Prioritize 7-9 hours of quality sleep each night. Sleep is when your body repairs and regenerates.

Active Recovery: Incorporate low-intensity activities like walking or gentle yoga on your rest days. This promotes circulation and aids in recovery.

Nutrition and Hydration: Continue to nourish your body with nutrient-rich foods and stay hydrated to support recovery.

Mindful Rest: Embrace mindfulness techniques, like meditation and deep breathing, to promote relaxation and reduce stress.

Adapting to Your Body's Feedback

As you engage in higher intensity workouts, it's essential to listen to your body's signals. Overtraining can lead to burnout and injury, so pay attention to signs of fatigue, soreness, or lack of motivation.

- Rest Days: Plan regular rest days to allow your body to recover and recharge.

- Modify Intensity: If a workout feels too challenging, don't hesitate to modify the intensity or switch to a lower impact activity.

- Incorporate Variety: Keep your workouts diverse to prevent overuse injuries and maintain motivation.

Tracking Progress and Celebrating Wins

During this intense phase, tracking your progress becomes even more vital. Celebrate each achievement, whether it's an increased weight lifted, improved endurance, or enhanced flexibility. Progress is not always linear, but tracking helps you see how far you've come.

Visual Progress: Take regular photos to visually document changes in your physique.

Strength Metrics: Keep a record of the weights, repetitions, and sets you're lifting. This helps you track improvements.

Endurance Benchmarks: Note the duration and intensity of your cardio workouts. Over time, you'll see your endurance soar.

In conclusion, the Day 31-45 phase of your fitness journey is all about embracing higher intensity workouts to cultivate power and endurance. With circuit training, interval workouts, and progressive resistance techniques, you're challenging your body to adapt and excel. Amidst this intensity, rest and recovery stand as pillars of progress, ensuring that your body can thrive under the demands placed upon it. As you navigate this phase, remember that every workout completed and every moment of self-care is an investment in your long-term strength, endurance, and well-being. Stay determined, stay adaptable, and let the power of this phase fuel your journey towards transformation.

CHAPTER SEVEN

Sustaining the Transformation: Day 46-60 and Beyond

As you approach the final phase of your 60-day fitness journey, a remarkable transformation has taken place. However, the journey doesn't end here—it transitions into a new chapter of sustaining the progress you've worked diligently to achieve. This chapter is a guide to navigating the Day 46-60 phase and beyond, focusing on consolidating your gains, embracing healthy habits, and transitioning into a sustainable lifestyle that maintains your hard-earned results. With guidance on modifying workouts, making healthy eating a habit, and crafting a personalized post-program fitness plan, you'll lay the foundation for a lifetime of wellness.

Consolidating Progress: A Lifestyle Shift

As you enter the final phase of the program, the goal is to solidify the progress you've made and transition from a structured fitness plan to a sustainable lifestyle. This shift involves:

Modifying Workouts for Long-Term Sustainability

Your fitness routine should evolve to meet your changing needs and goals. Consider these modifications:

- Variety: Introduce new exercises, routines, and activities to keep your workouts engaging.

- Frequency: Gradually reduce the frequency of high-intensity workouts while incorporating more recovery days.

- Strength and Cardio Balance: Shift your focus from intense cardio to maintaining a balance between cardiovascular exercise and strength training.

Incorporating Movement Into Your Day

Embrace a more active lifestyle by incorporating movement into your daily routine:

- Walk More: Aim for at least 10,000 steps a day. Walking is a low-impact way to maintain cardiovascular health.

- Active Commuting: If feasible, bike or walk to work instead of driving.

- Micro Workouts: Sneak in short bursts of exercise throughout the day—push-ups, squats, or stretching.

Making Healthy Eating a Habit

Healthy eating is not just a short-term endeavor—it's a lifelong habit that supports your fitness and well-being. Focus on these principles:

- Balance: Continue to prioritize a balanced intake of protein, carbohydrates, and healthy fats.

- Mindful Eating: Pay attention to hunger and fullness cues to prevent overeating.

- Nutrient Density: Choose nutrient-rich foods like fruits, vegetables, whole grains, and lean proteins.

- Moderation: Allow yourself occasional treats while maintaining an overall healthy eating pattern.

Crafting a Personalized Post-Program Fitness Plan

Your journey doesn't conclude after Day 60—it evolves. Create a personalized fitness plan that aligns with your goals, preferences, and lifestyle:

- Set New Goals: Whether it's running a 10K, achieving a specific strength milestone, or improving flexibility, having new goals keeps you motivated.

- Mix It Up: Explore different types of workouts and activities to prevent boredom and plateaus.

- Long-Term Sustainability: Design your plan with longevity in mind. Avoid extreme measures that are difficult to maintain.

- Consistency: Aim for consistent workouts and healthy eating habits, even if they're at a lower intensity than during the program.

Mindset: The Key to Long-Term Success

A positive and adaptable mindset is the linchpin of sustaining your transformation. Embrace the following principles:

- Celebrate Non-Scale Victories: Shift your focus from just the numbers on the scale to other achievements like increased energy, improved mood, and enhanced confidence.

- Self-Compassion: Be kind to yourself during setbacks. Accept that progress may not always be linear.

- Embrace Flexibility: Life is dynamic, and your fitness journey should be too. Be willing to adjust your plan as circumstances change.

Community and Support

The journey is often more enjoyable and successful when shared with others:

- Accountability Partners: Team up with a friend or family member to keep each other motivated and accountable.

- Online Communities: Join fitness forums or social media groups to connect with like-minded individuals.

- Professional Support: Consider working with a fitness coach or nutritionist to receive expert guidance tailored to your needs.

Mind and Body Wellness

Remember that fitness is not just about physical transformation—it's about holistic well-being.

Prioritize mental health, sleep, and stress reduction:

- Mindfulness Practices: Continue practicing meditation, visualization, and stress reduction techniques to support mental well-being.

- Quality Sleep: Prioritize sleep for recovery, energy, and cognitive function.

- Stress Management: Incorporate stress reduction techniques to prevent burnout and promote overall balance.

Reflecting on Your Journey

As you approach the conclusion of your 60-day program, take time to reflect on your achievements:

- Journaling: Write about your progress, challenges, and how you've grown physically and mentally.

- Before and After: Compare your initial photos and measurements with your current ones to see the tangible changes.

- Gratitude: Express gratitude for your body's capabilities and the dedication you've shown to your well-being.

Transitioning Beyond Day 60

The 60-day program is a stepping stone into a lifelong journey of health and fitness. Remember that transformation is ongoing:

- Set New Goals: Continue to set and achieve new fitness goals to maintain motivation and growth.

- Reassess and Adjust: Regularly reassess your fitness plan to ensure it aligns with your evolving goals and needs.

- Listen to Your Body: Pay attention to how your body responds to different exercises and adjust accordingly.

- Enjoy the Journey: Relish in the process of living a healthier, more active life. Embrace challenges as opportunities for growth.

In conclusion, the Day 46-60 phase of your fitness journey marks a transition from structured workouts to a sustainable lifestyle. By modifying workouts, embracing healthy eating as a habit, and crafting a personalized post-program fitness plan, you're setting the stage for lasting success. A positive mindset, community support, and holistic wellness practices further enrich your journey. As you embark on this final stretch and beyond, remember that the transformation you've achieved is not just physical—it's a testament to your dedication, resilience, and commitment to lifelong well-being. Celebrate every step you've taken and those that lie ahead, knowing that your journey towards health and vitality is a continuous and rewarding adventure.